A Guide To Understanding Acetaminophen

The Comprehensive Guidebook to understand how acetaminophen works

Mathilda West

Contents

Chapter1 3
  Introduction to Acetaminophen 3
Chapter2 15
  Dosage of acetaminophen 15
Chapter3 26
  Side effects of acetaminophen 26
Chapter4 38
  Acetaminophen precautions and warnings 38
The end 57

Chapter 1

Introduction to Acetaminophen

Acetaminophen, also known as paracetamol, is a widely used over-the-counter medication primarily utilized for its analgesic (pain-relieving) and antipyretic (fever-reducing) properties. Here's an overview of its key aspects:

Chemical Properties:

- **Chemical Name:** N-(4-hydroxyphenyl)acetamide

- **Molecular Formula:** $C_8H_9NO_2$

- **Molecular Weight:** 151.16 g/mol

Mechanism of Action:

Acetaminophen works by inhibiting the synthesis of prostaglandins in the brain, which are chemicals that promote inflammation, pain, and fever. Unlike nonsteroidal anti-inflammatory drugs (NSAIDs) such as ibuprofen and aspirin, acetaminophen does not have significant anti-inflammatory properties.

Uses:

1. **Pain Relief:** Effective for mild to moderate pain such

as headaches, muscle aches, menstrual periods, toothaches, and backaches.

2. **Fever Reduction:** Helps in reducing fever in adults and children.

Dosage:

- **Adults:** The typical dose is 500 to 1000 mg every 4 to 6 hours as needed, not exceeding 4000 mg in 24 hours.

- **Children:** Dosage varies based on weight and age, so it's crucial to follow the guidelines provided by a healthcare professional or the product label.

Side Effects:

- Generally well-tolerated when used at recommended doses.

- Possible side effects include nausea, rash, and headache.

- Overdose can lead to severe liver damage, which can be fatal. Symptoms of overdose include nausea, vomiting, sweating, and confusion.

Precautions:

- Avoid consuming alcohol while taking acetaminophen, as

this increases the risk of liver damage.

- Be cautious when using other medications that contain acetaminophen to avoid exceeding the recommended daily dose.

Interactions:

- Acetaminophen can interact with other medications such as warfarin (a blood thinner), potentially increasing the risk of bleeding.
- It's essential to check with a healthcare provider before combining it with other drugs.

Conclusion:

Acetaminophen is a valuable medication for managing pain and fever when used correctly. It's important to adhere to the recommended dosages and be aware of potential risks, especially concerning liver health. For any questions or concerns regarding its use, consulting with a healthcare professional is advisable.

Chapter 2

Dosage of acetaminophen For Adults:

1. **Standard Dose:**

   - **Regular Strength (325 mg tablets):** 1-2 tablets every 4 to 6 hours as needed. Do not exceed 10 tablets (3250 mg) in 24 hours.

- **Extra Strength (500 mg tablets):** 1-2 tablets every 6 hours as needed. Do not exceed 6 tablets (3000 mg) in 24 hours.

- **Extended-Release (650 mg tablets):** 1-2 tablets every 8 hours as needed. Do not exceed 6 tablets (3900 mg) in 24 hours.

2. **Maximum Dose:**

- **General Limit:** Do not exceed 4000 mg in 24 hours.
- **Recommended Lower Limit:** Many healthcare providers recommend not exceeding 3000 mg per day to minimize the

risk of liver damage.

For Children:

- **Infants and Children Under 2 Years:**
    - Dosage should be determined by a healthcare provider.

- **Children 2 to 12 Years:**
  - **Liquid Suspension (160 mg/5 mL):** The dosage is based on the child's weight.
  - **Weight-Based Dosage:**

- 24-35 lbs (2-3 years): 5 mL (160 mg) every 4 to 6 hours as needed. Do not exceed 5 doses (800 mg) in 24 hours.
- 36-47 lbs (4-5 years): 7.5

mL (240 mg) every 4 to 6 hours as needed. Do not exceed 5 doses (1200 mg) in 24 hours.

- 48-59 lbs (6-8 years): 10 mL (320 mg) every 4 to 6

hours as needed. Do not exceed 5 doses (1600 mg) in 24 hours.

- 60-71 lbs (9-10 years): 12.5 mL (400 mg) every 4 to 6 hours as needed. Do not exceed 5 doses (2000 mg) in 24 hours.

- 72-95 lbs (11 years): 15 mL (480 mg) every 4 to 6 hours as needed. Do not exceed 5 doses (2400 mg) in 24 hours.

Chapter 3

Side effects of acetaminophen

Common Side Effects:

- **Nausea**

- **Vomiting**

- **Headache**

- **Rash**

These side effects are usually mild and

temporary. If they persist or worsen, it's important to contact a healthcare provider.

Serious Side Effects:

Though rare, serious side effects can occur, especially with overdose or prolonged use. These include:

- **Liver Damage:**

- Symptoms: Jaundice (yellowing of the skin/eyes), dark urine, fatigue, nausea, vomiting, loss of appetite.
- Risk increases with excessive dosing or

combining with alcohol.

- **Severe Allergic Reactions (Anaphylaxis):**
  - Symptoms: Difficulty breathing, swelling of the face/lips/tongue/throat, severe

rash, itching, dizziness.
  - This is a medical emergency and requires immediate attention.
- **Stevens-Johnson Syndrome (SJS) and Toxic Epidermal Necrolysis (TEN):**

- Symptoms: Severe skin rash, blistering, peeling of the skin, sores in the mouth, nose, eyes, or genital area.
- These are rare but serious conditions that require

immediate medical attention.

- **Kidney Damage:**
  - Symptoms: Changes in urine output, swelling of the legs or ankles, fatigue.

- More likely with prolonged use or high doses.

Signs of Overdose:

Acetaminophen overdose is a medical emergency and can lead to severe liver damage or failure. Symptoms of overdose include:

- Nausea
- Vomiting
- Loss of appetite
- Sweating
- Confusion
- Weakness
- Stomach pain
- Yellowing of the skin or eyes (jaundice)

If an overdose is suspected, seek emergency medical attention immediately or contact a poison control center.

Precautions:

- **Alcohol Consumption:** Avoid alcohol while taking acetaminophen to reduce the risk of liver damage.

- **Pre-existing Conditions:** Inform your healthcare provider if you have liver disease, kidney disease, or a history of alcohol abuse.

- **Medication Interactions:** Be cautious about

taking other medications that contain acetaminophen to avoid unintentional overdose. Check labels and consult a healthcare provider

Chapter 4

Acetaminophen precautions and warnings

General Precautions:

1. **Dosage Adherence:**

    ○ Do not exceed the recommended dose. Taking more than the

recommended amount can cause serious liver damage.

2. **Read Labels Carefully:**

- Acetaminophen is a common ingredient in many over-the-counter and prescription medications, including pain relievers, fever reducers, and cold and flu medications. Ensure you are not taking multiple products containing acetaminophen simultaneously.

3. **Consult Healthcare Providers:**

   - Always consult with a healthcare provider before taking acetaminophen if you have any existing health conditions or are taking other medications.

Specific Warnings:

1. **Liver Damage:**
   - High doses or prolonged use of acetaminophen can lead to liver damage or

failure. The risk is higher if you consume alcohol regularly or have pre-existing liver conditions.

- Avoid alcohol while taking acetaminophen.

2. **Allergic Reactions:**

- Severe allergic reactions, such as anaphylaxis, are rare but possible. Symptoms include swelling of the face, lips, tongue, or throat, severe rash, itching, dizziness, and difficulty breathing. Seek immediate medical attention if you experience these symptoms.

3. **Skin Reactions:**
   - Rare but serious skin reactions such as

Stevens-Johnson Syndrome (SJS) and Toxic Epidermal Necrolysis (TEN) can occur. Symptoms include severe rash, blistering, peeling of the skin, and sores in the mouth, nose, eyes, or genital area. These require immediate medical attention.

4. **Kidney Damage:**

    - Prolonged use or high doses may lead to kidney damage.

Symptoms include changes in urine output, swelling of the legs or ankles, and fatigue. Consult a healthcare provider if you experience these symptoms.

5. **Chronic Use:**

- Long-term use, even at recommended doses, can increase the risk of liver and kidney damage. Discuss with a healthcare provider before using acetaminophen for extended periods.

Special Populations:

1. **Pregnant and Breastfeeding Women:**

    - Acetaminophen is generally considered safe during pregnancy and breastfeeding when used as directed. However, it is important to consult a healthcare provider before use.

2. **Children:**

    ◦ Dosage for children should

be determined based on weight and age. Always follow the guidelines provided by a healthcare professional or the product label.

3. **Older Adults:**

- Older adults may be more susceptible to the side effects of acetaminophen. Lower doses may be recommended.

Interactions with Other Medications:

1. **Blood Thinners (e.g., Warfarin):**
   - Acetaminophen can interact with blood thinners, increasing the risk of bleeding. Consult a healthcare provider before using acetaminophen

if you are on blood thinners.

2. **Other Pain Relievers:**

- Avoid combining acetaminophen with other pain relievers, especially those containing acetaminophen, to prevent overdose.

The end

www.ingramcontent.com/pod-product-compliance
Lightning Source LLC
Chambersburg PA
CBHW071844210526
45479CB00001B/280